DIABETIC KIDNEY-FRIENDLY MEAL PLANS

PLANS

Easy, Delicious Recipes for Managing Your Health

Dr Lily Morgan

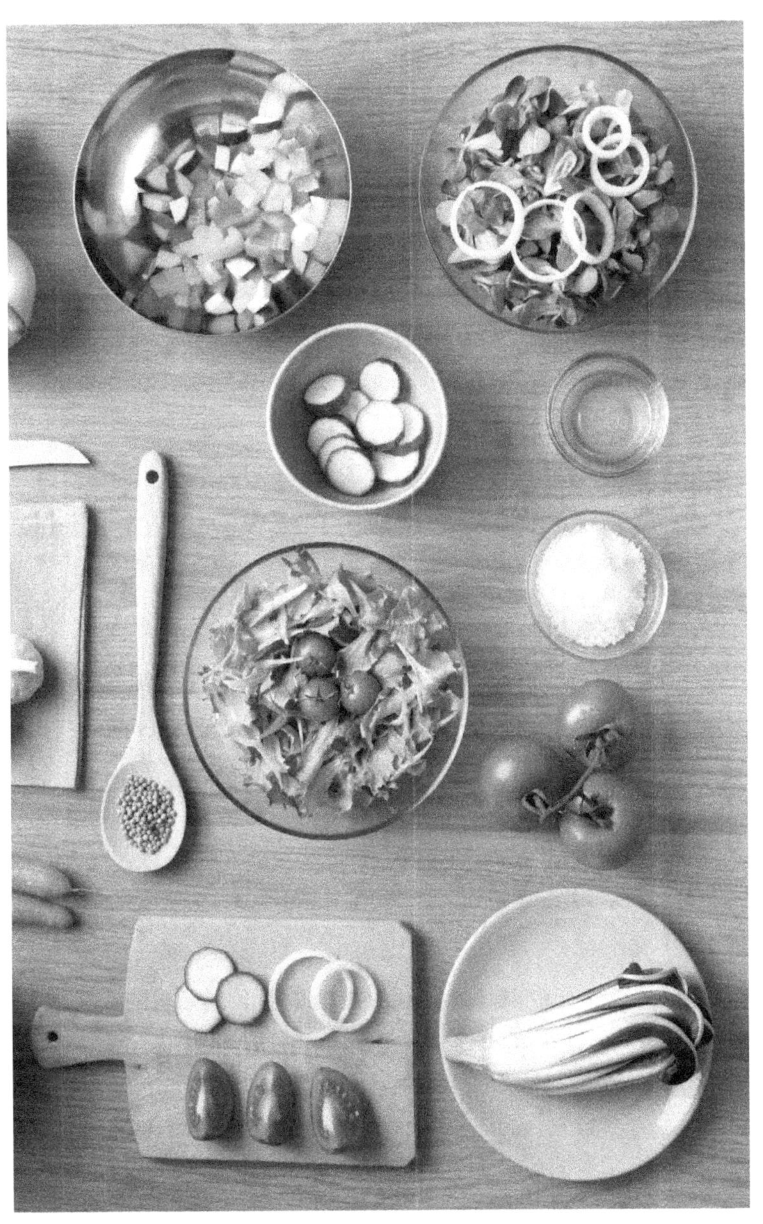

TABLE OF CONTENTS

Chapter 5: Snacks and Appetizers 72

INTRODUCTION

In our journey towards a healthier, more fulfilling life, understanding the intricacies of diabetic kidney-friendly meal planning is a fundamental step. This process isn't just about managing diabetes; it's a holistic approach that prioritizes the well-being of your kidneys, a vital but often underappreciated part of our bodies.

When it comes to managing diabetes, the importance of nutrition cannot be overstated. It's not merely about counting carbs or monitoring blood sugar levels; it's about nourishing your body in a way that supports your kidneys. These vital organs work tirelessly to filter waste and excess fluids from our blood, ensuring our internal environment remains in balance. However, for those with diabetes, the kidneys can face additional stress.

Diabetic kidney health is an intricate dance of nutrition and careful choices. Meal planning becomes an art, with each dish carefully composed to harmonize with your dietary needs. By paying attention to the nutritional content of what we consume, we can make life easier for our kidneys. But it's not just about limiting certain elements; it's also about embracing the right ones.

High-quality protein sources, such as lean meats, fish, and plant-based options, can play a pivotal role in supporting your kidney health. A diet rich in whole grains, fresh fruits, and vegetables provides essential vitamins and minerals while maintaining steady blood sugar levels. These ingredients act as the building blocks of a diabetic kidney-friendly meal plan, ensuring that your nutrition aligns with your health goals.

Beyond the physical aspects, it's essential to understand the emotional and psychological aspects of this journey. The choices we make about what we eat can be both empowering and emotionally nourishing. Diabetic kidney-friendly meal planning isn't a limitation; it's an opportunity for creativity, exploration, and renewal.

The impact of a well-thought-out meal plan extends far beyond the dining table. It ripples through your daily life, influencing your energy levels, mood, and overall vitality. When you prioritize nutrition for diabetic kidney health, you're taking control of your well-being in the most meaningful way.

So, as you embark on this journey of understanding diabetic kidney-friendly meal planning, remember that it's not just about what's on your plate; it's about what's in your life. It's a path towards a healthier, more fulfilling existence, where nutrition is not just a duty but a celebration of your health and your kidneys' invaluable work.

Chapter 1: 30-Day Meal Plan

Week 1:

Day 1

- Breakfast: Low-Sugar Berry Smoothie
- Lunch: Turkey and Avocado Wrap
- Dinner: Grilled Salmon with Lemon-Dill Sauce
- Snack: Mixed Nuts
- Dessert: Sugar-Free Berry Sorbet

Day 2

- Breakfast: Veggie Omelette with Spinach
- Lunch: Quinoa and Chickpea Salad
- Dinner: Baked Chicken Breast with Asparagus
- Snack: Greek Yogurt and Berries
- Dessert: Chocolate Avocado Pudding

Day 3

- Breakfast: Avocado and Turkey Breakfast Wrap
- Lunch: Grilled Chicken Salad with Balsamic Vinaigrette

- Dinner: Spaghetti Squash with Tomato Sauce
- Snack: Hummus and Veggies
- Dessert: Baked Apple with Cinnamon

Day 4

- Breakfast: Greek Yogurt Parfait
- Lunch: Lentil Soup
- Dinner: Shrimp and Vegetable Skewers
- Snack: Cottage Cheese with Pineapple
- Dessert: Greek Yogurt Parfait with Honey

Day 5

- Breakfast: Cinnamon Oatmeal with Walnuts
- Lunch: Tuna Salad Lettuce Wraps
- Dinner: Black Bean and Quinoa Stuffed Peppers
- Snack: Stuffed Bell Pepper Poppers
- Dessert: Frozen Banana Bites

Day 6

- Breakfast: Whole Grain Pancakes
- Lunch: Spinach and Quinoa Stuffed Peppers
- Dinner: Garlic and Herb Roasted Turkey

- Snack: Guacamole with Veggie Sticks
- Dessert: Chia Seed Chocolate Pudding

Day 7

- Breakfast: Sweet Potato and Black Bean Hash
- Lunch: Chicken and Vegetable Stir-Fry
- Dinner: Tofu and Vegetable Stir-Fry
- Snack: Hard-Boiled Eggs
- Dessert: Berry and Almond Tart

Week 2:

Day 8

- Breakfast: Quinoa Breakfast Bowl
- Lunch: Greek Salad with Grilled Chicken
- Dinner: Baked Cod with Herb Crust
- Snack: Caprese Skewers
- Dessert: Oatmeal Raisin Cookies (Sugar-Free)

Day 9

- Breakfast: Scrambled Eggs with Spinach and Feta
- Lunch: Veggie and Hummus Wrap
- Dinner: Stuffed Zucchini Boats

- Snack: Cucumber Slices with Tzatziki
- Dessert: Pumpkin Pie Smoothie

Day 10

- Breakfast: Chia Seed Pudding
- Lunch: Bean and Vegetable Chili
- Dinner: Turkey and Vegetable Curry
- Snack: Edamame
- Dessert: Lemon Blueberry Muffins (Sugar-Free)

Day 11

- Breakfast: Breakfast Quiche with Zucchini
- Lunch: Turkey and Vegetable Stir-Fry
- Dinner: Eggplant and Tomato Bake
- Snack: Apple Slices with Almond Butter
- Dessert: Almond and Coconut Bites

Day 12

- Breakfast: Peanut Butter and Banana Toast
- Lunch: Spinach and Mushroom Quesadilla
- Dinner: Lemon Herb Tilapia
- Snack: Mini Turkey Lettuce Wraps

- Dessert: Avocado Chocolate Mousse

Day 13

- Breakfast: Vegetable Frittata
- Lunch: Cucumber and Chickpea Salad
- Dinner: Butternut Squash and Chickpea Stew
- Snack: Popcorn with Nutritional Yeast
- Dessert: Peach and Raspberry Crumble

Day 14

- Breakfast: Blueberry Almond Overnight Oats
- Lunch: Sweet Potato and Black Bean Salad
- Dinner: Beef and Vegetable Stir-Fry
- Snack: Roasted Chickpeas
- Dessert: Rice Pudding with Cinnamon

Week 3:

Day 15

- Breakfast: Strawberry Cheesecake Bites
- Lunch: Zucchini Noodle Salad with Pesto
- Dinner: Mushroom and Spinach Stuffed Chicken
- Snack: Mini Caprese Salad

- Dessert: Strawberry Cheesecake Bites

Day 16

- Breakfast: Carrot Cake Bites
- Lunch: Egg Salad Lettuce Wraps
- Dinner: Cilantro Lime Shrimp
- Snack: Sliced Bell Peppers with Peanut Butter
- Dessert: Carrot Cake Bites

Day 17

- Breakfast: Apple Cinnamon Baked Oatmeal
- Lunch: Caprese Salad with Balsamic Glaze
- Dinner: Baked Sweet Potato Fries
- Snack: Baked Sweet Potato Fries
- Dessert: Apple Cinnamon Baked Oatmeal

Day 18

- Breakfast: Rice Cake with Cottage Cheese and Berries
- Lunch: Greek Salad with Grilled Chicken
- Dinner: Baked Cod with Herb Crust
- Snack: Mixed Nuts

- Dessert: Sugar-Free Berry Sorbet

Day 19

- Breakfast: Oat Bran Muffins
- Lunch: Veggie and Hummus Wrap
- Dinner: Stuffed Zucchini Boats
- Snack: Greek Yogurt and Berries
- Dessert: Chocolate Avocado Pudding

Day 20

- Breakfast: Tofu and Vegetable Scramble
- Lunch: Bean and Vegetable Chili
- Dinner: Turkey and Vegetable Curry
- Snack: Cottage Cheese with Pineapple
- Dessert: Greek Yogurt Parfait with Honey

Day 21

- Breakfast: Stuffed Bell Pepper Poppers
- Lunch: Chicken and Vegetable Stir-Fry
- Dinner: Lemon Herb Tilapia
- Snack: Guacamole with Veggie Sticks
- Dessert: Baked Apple with Cinnamon

Week 4:

Day 22

- Breakfast: Peanut Butter and Banana Toast
- Lunch: Spinach and Mushroom Quesadilla
- Dinner: Butternut Squash and Chickpea Stew
- Snack: Hard-Boiled Eggs
- Dessert: Lemon Blueberry Muffins (Sugar-Free)

Day 23

- Breakfast: Vegetable Frittata
- Lunch: Cucumber and Chickpea Salad
- Dinner: Beef and Vegetable Stir-Fry
- Snack: Edamame
- Dessert: Almond and Coconut Bites

Day 24

- Breakfast: Blueberry Almond Overnight Oats
- Lunch: Sweet Potato and Black Bean Salad
- Dinner: Mushroom and Spinach Stuffed Chicken
- Snack: Roasted Chickpeas
- Dessert: Avocado Chocolate Mousse

Day 25

- Breakfast: Strawberry Cheesecake Bites
- Lunch: Zucchini Noodle Salad with Pesto
- Dinner: Cilantro Lime Shrimp
- Snack: Mini Caprese Salad
- Dessert: Strawberry Cheesecake Bites

Day 26

- Breakfast: Carrot Cake Bites
- Lunch: Egg Salad Lettuce Wraps
- Dinner: Cabbage and Sausage Skillet
- Snack: Sliced Bell Peppers with Peanut Butter
- Dessert: Carrot Cake Bites

Day 27

- Breakfast: Apple Cinnamon Baked Oatmeal
- Lunch: Caprese Salad with Balsamic Glaze
- Dinner: Baked Sweet Potato Fries
- Snack: Baked Sweet Potato Fries
- Dessert: Apple Cinnamon Baked Oatmeal

Day 28

- Breakfast: Rice Cake with Cottage Cheese and Berries
- Lunch: Greek Salad with Grilled Chicken
- Dinner: Baked Cod with Herb Crust
- Snack: Mixed Nuts
- Dessert: Sugar-Free Berry Sorbet

Day 29

- Breakfast: Oat Bran Muffins
- Lunch: Veggie and Hummus Wrap
- Dinner: Stuffed Zucchini Boats
- Snack: Greek Yogurt and Berries
- Dessert: Chocolate Avocado Pudding

Day 30

- Breakfast: Tofu and Vegetable Scramble
- Lunch: Bean and Vegetable Chili
- Dinner: Turkey and Vegetable Curry
- Snack: Cottage Cheese with Pineapple
- Dessert: Greek Yogurt Parfait with Honey

This 30-day meal plan offers a diverse range of delicious and kidney-friendly recipes for each day. Enjoy your meals!

Chapter 2: Breakfast Recipes

In this chapter, we embark on a culinary journey to craft a collection of breakfast recipes that harmoniously blend flavor, nutrition, and simplicity. These recipes are thoughtfully designed to cater to those seeking a diabetic and kidney-friendly start to their day.

Low-Sugar Berry Smoothie

Ingredients:

- 1 cup mixed berries (strawberries, blueberries, raspberries)
- 1/2 cup Greek yogurt
- 1 tablespoon chia seeds
- 1/2 cup unsweetened almond milk
- Ice cubes (optional)

Instructions:

1. Combine the berries, Greek yogurt, chia seeds, and almond milk in a blender.
2. Blend until smooth.

3. Add ice cubes if desired and blend again.

4. Pour into a glass and enjoy this refreshing low-sugar smoothie.

Veggie Omelette with Spinach

Ingredients:

- 2 eggs
- 1/4 cup spinach, chopped
- 1/4 cup red bell pepper, diced
- 1/4 cup onion, diced
- Salt and pepper to taste
- Cooking spray or a small amount of olive oil

Instructions:

1. In a bowl, beat the eggs and add a pinch of salt and pepper.

2. Heat a non-stick skillet and lightly coat it with cooking spray or olive oil.

3. Sauté the onions and bell pepper until tender, then add the chopped spinach.

4. Pour the beaten eggs over the veggies.

5. Cook until the omelette is set, then fold it in half and
serve.

Avocado and Turkey Breakfast Wrap

Ingredients:

- 1 whole-grain tortilla
- 1/2 avocado, sliced
- 2 slices of turkey breast
- 1/4 cup baby spinach
- 1 tablespoon Greek yogurt (optional)
- Salsa or hot sauce for extra flavor (optional)

Instructions:

1. Lay the tortilla flat and spread the avocado evenly.
2. Place turkey slices and baby spinach on top.
3. Optionally, add a dollop of Greek yogurt and a dash of salsa.
4. Roll the tortilla into a wrap and enjoy this wholesome breakfast.

Greek Yogurt Parfait

Ingredients:

- 1 cup Greek yogurt
- 1/2 cup mixed berries
- 2 tablespoons chopped nuts (almonds or walnuts)
- 1 teaspoon honey (optional)

Instructions:

1. In a glass or bowl, layer Greek yogurt, mixed berries, and chopped nuts.
2. Drizzle with honey if desired.
3. Savor the delightful combination of creamy yogurt, sweet berries, and crunchy nuts.

Cinnamon Oatmeal with Walnuts

Ingredients:

- 1/2 cup rolled oats
- 1 cup water or almond milk
- 1/2 teaspoon ground cinnamon
- 1 tablespoon chopped walnuts
- 1/2 small banana, sliced

Instructions:

1. In a saucepan, combine oats, water or almond milk, and cinnamon.

2. Cook on medium heat, stirring occasionally, until the oats are soft and creamy.

3. Serve with chopped walnuts and banana slices for added texture and natural sweetness.

Whole Grain Pancakes

Ingredients:

- 1/2 cup whole wheat flour
- 1/2 teaspoon baking powder
- 1/4 teaspoon salt
- 1/2 cup unsweetened almond milk
- 1 egg
- 1/2 teaspoon vanilla extract
- Cooking spray or a small amount of olive oil

Instructions:

1. In a bowl, mix whole wheat flour, baking powder, and salt.

2. In another bowl, whisk almond milk, egg, and vanilla extract.

3. Combine the wet and dry ingredients.

4. Heat a non-stick skillet and coat it with cooking spray or olive oil.

5. Pour the pancake batter onto the skillet and cook until golden brown on both sides.

6. Serve these hearty whole grain pancakes with your favorite toppings.

Sweet Potato and Black Bean Hash

Ingredients:

- 1 small sweet potato, diced
- 1/2 cup black beans, cooked and drained
- 1/4 cup red bell pepper, diced
- 1/4 cup onion, diced
- 1/2 teaspoon cumin
- Salt and pepper to taste
- Cooking spray or a small amount of olive oil

Instructions:

1. Heat a skillet and lightly coat it with cooking spray or olive oil.

2. Sauté the diced sweet potato, red bell pepper, and onion until they are tender.

3. Add the cooked black beans, cumin, salt, and pepper.

4. Continue cooking until everything is heated through and slightly crispy.

Quinoa Breakfast Bowl

Ingredients:

- 1/2 cup cooked quinoa
- 1/4 cup unsweetened almond milk
- 1/4 cup mixed berries
- 1 tablespoon chopped nuts (e.g., almonds or pecans)
- 1/2 teaspoon honey (optional)

Instructions:

1. In a bowl, combine cooked quinoa and almond milk.

2. Top with mixed berries and chopped nuts.

3. Drizzle with honey if desired.

4. This quinoa bowl provides a nutritious and energizing start to your day.

Scrambled Eggs with Spinach and Feta

Ingredients:

- 2 eggs
- 1/2 cup fresh spinach, chopped
- 2 tablespoons crumbled feta cheese
- Salt and pepper to taste
- Cooking spray or a small amount of olive oil

Instructions:

1. In a bowl, beat the eggs and season with salt and pepper.
2. Heat a skillet and lightly coat it with cooking spray or olive oil.
3. Add chopped spinach and sauté until wilted.
4. Pour in the beaten eggs and cook, stirring gently, until they're scrambled.
5. Sprinkle feta cheese over the eggs and serve.

Chia Seed Pudding

Ingredients:

- 2 tablespoons chia seeds
- 1/2 cup unsweetened almond milk
- 1/2 teaspoon vanilla extract
- 1/2 cup mixed berries
- 1 teaspoon honey (optional)

Instructions:

1. In a container, mix chia seeds, almond milk, and vanilla extract.
2. Stir well and refrigerate for at least 2 hours or overnight until it thickens.
3. Serve with mixed berries and a drizzle of honey if you prefer a touch of sweetness.

Breakfast Quiche with Zucchini

Ingredients:

- 4 eggs
- 1/2 cup zucchini, grated
- 1/4 cup red bell pepper, diced

- 1/4 cup onion, diced
- 2 tablespoons grated Parmesan cheese
- Salt and pepper to taste
- Cooking spray or a small amount of olive oil

Instructions:

1. Preheat your oven to 350°F (175°C).
2. In a bowl, beat the eggs and add grated zucchini, red bell pepper, onion, Parmesan cheese, salt, and pepper.
3. Pour the mixture into a greased muffin tin or quiche dish.
4. Bake for 25-30 minutes or until the quiche is set and slightly browned.

Peanut Butter and Banana Toast

Ingredients:

- 1 slice of whole-grain bread
- 1 tablespoon natural peanut butter
- 1/2 banana, sliced

Instructions:

1. Toast the whole-grain bread to your desired level of crispness.

2. Spread a layer of natural peanut butter on the toast.

3. Arrange banana slices on top for a delightful combination of flavors and textures.

Vegetable Frittata

Ingredients:

- 4 eggs
- 1/4 cup bell peppers, diced
- 1/4 cup zucchini, diced
- 1/4 cup cherry tomatoes, halved
- 2 tablespoons feta cheese
- Salt and pepper to taste
- Cooking spray or a small amount of olive oil

Instructions:

1. Preheat your oven to 350°F (175°C).

2. In a bowl, beat the eggs and season with salt and pepper.

3. Heat an oven-safe skillet, coat it with cooking spray or olive oil, and sauté the diced vegetables.

4. Pour the beaten eggs over the vegetables, sprinkle with feta cheese, and cook for a few minutes.

5. Transfer the skillet to the oven and bake for about 10 minutes or until the frittata is set.

Blueberry Almond Overnight Oats

Ingredients:

- 1/2 cup rolled oats
- 1/2 cup unsweetened almond milk
- 1/4 cup blueberries
- 1 tablespoon sliced almonds
- 1/2 teaspoon vanilla extract

Instructions:

1. In a jar or container, combine oats, almond milk, blueberries, sliced almonds, and vanilla extract.

2. Stir well and refrigerate overnight.

3. Enjoy these creamy, no-cook overnight oats in the morning.

Breakfast Burrito

Ingredients:

- 1 whole-grain tortilla
- 2 eggs, scrambled
- 1/4 cup black beans, cooked and drained
- 1/4 cup diced tomatoes
- 1/4 cup diced onions
- 1/4 cup shredded low-fat cheese (optional)
- Salsa or hot sauce for extra flavor (optional)

Instructions:

1. Lay the tortilla flat and add scrambled eggs, black beans, tomatoes, onions, and cheese if desired.
2. Optionally, add salsa or hot sauce for an extra kick of flavor.
3. Roll up the tortilla into a burrito and enjoy this savory and satisfying breakfast.

Rice Cake with Cottage Cheese and Berries

Ingredients:

- 1 rice cake
- 1/4 cup low-fat cottage cheese
- 1/4 cup mixed berries

Instructions:

1. Spread low-fat cottage cheese on the rice cake.
2. Top with mixed berries for a light and refreshing breakfast.

Oat Bran Muffins

Ingredients:

- 1 cup oat bran
- 1/4 cup unsweetened applesauce
- 1/4 cup almond milk
- 2 eggs
- 2 tablespoons honey
- 1/2 teaspoon cinnamon
- 1/2 teaspoon baking powder

Instructions:

1. Preheat your oven to 350°F (175°C) and line a muffin tin with paper liners.
2. In a bowl, combine oat bran, applesauce, almond milk, eggs, honey, cinnamon, and baking powder.
3. Mix well and pour the batter into the muffin tin.
4. Bake for 20-25 minutes or until the muffins are firm and slightly browned.

Tofu and Vegetable Scramble

Ingredients:

- 1/2 cup firm tofu, crumbled
- 1/4 cup bell peppers, diced
- 1/4 cup spinach, chopped
- 1/4 cup cherry tomatoes, halved
- 1/4 cup onion, diced
- 1/2 teaspoon turmeric
- Salt and pepper to taste
- Cooking spray or a small amount of olive oil

Instructions:

1. Heat a skillet and lightly coat it with cooking spray or olive oil.

2. Sauté diced vegetables until tender.

3. Add crumbled tofu, turmeric, salt, and pepper.

4. Cook until the tofu is heated through and slightly golden.

Chapter 3: Lunch Recipes

In this chapter, you'll find a delightful array of lunch recipes that are not only delicious but also perfect for those managing their diabetic and kidney health. Each recipe is thoughtfully crafted to provide a burst of flavors while keeping nutrition in focus. Let's embark on this culinary journey that combines taste and well-being.

Turkey and Avocado Wrap

Ingredients:

- 4 large whole-grain tortillas
- 8 ounces sliced turkey breast
- 1 ripe avocado, sliced
- 1 cup lettuce leaves
- 1/4 cup low-fat mayonnaise
- 1 teaspoon Dijon mustard
- Salt and pepper to taste

Instructions:

1. Lay out a tortilla.

2. Spread a thin layer of mayonnaise and Dijon mustard on it.

3. Layer turkey slices, avocado, and lettuce.

4. Season with salt and pepper.

5. Roll the tortilla tightly, cut in half, and enjoy.

Quinoa and Chickpea Salad

Ingredients:

- 1 cup quinoa, cooked and cooled
- 1 can chickpeas, drained and rinsed
- 1 cup cherry tomatoes, halved
- 1 cucumber, diced
- 1/4 cup red onion, finely chopped
- 1/4 cup fresh parsley, chopped
- 2 tablespoons olive oil
- 2 tablespoons lemon juice
- Salt and pepper to taste

Instructions:

1. In a large bowl, combine quinoa, chickpeas, cherry tomatoes, cucumber, red onion, and parsley.

2. In a small bowl, whisk together olive oil and lemon juice.

3. Pour the dressing over the salad and toss to combine.

4. Season with salt and pepper.

5. Chill before serving.

Grilled Chicken Salad with Balsamic Vinaigrette

Ingredients:

- 2 boneless, skinless chicken breasts
- 6 cups mixed greens
- 1 cup cherry tomatoes, halved
- 1/2 red onion, thinly sliced
- 1/4 cup balsamic vinaigrette dressing
- 2 tablespoons olive oil
- Salt and pepper to taste

Instructions:

1. Preheat a grill or grill pan over medium-high heat.

2. Season chicken breasts with salt and pepper.

3. Grill chicken until cooked through, about 6-7 minutes per side.

4. Let the chicken rest for a few minutes, then slice it.

5. In a large bowl, combine mixed greens, cherry tomatoes, and red onion.

6. Drizzle with balsamic vinaigrette and olive oil.

7. Toss to coat.

8. Top with sliced chicken.

Lentil Soup

Ingredients:

- 1 cup green or brown lentils
- 1 onion, chopped
- 2 carrots, diced
- 2 celery stalks, diced
- 3 cloves garlic, minced
- 6 cups low-sodium vegetable broth
- 1 teaspoon cumin
- 1 teaspoon paprika
- Salt and pepper to taste

Instructions:

1. In a large pot, sauté onions, carrots, celery, and garlic until softened.
2. Add lentils, vegetable broth, cumin, and paprika.
3. Bring to a boil, then reduce heat and simmer for 30-35 minutes.
4. Season with salt and pepper.
5. Serve hot.

Tuna Salad Lettuce Wraps

Ingredients:

- 2 cans tuna in water, drained
- 1/4 cup plain Greek yogurt
- 1/4 cup diced celery
- 1/4 cup diced red onion
- 1 tablespoon lemon juice
- Salt and pepper to taste
- Lettuce leaves for wrapping

Instructions:

1. In a bowl, combine tuna, Greek yogurt, celery, red onion, and lemon juice.

2. Mix well and season with salt and pepper.

3. Spoon the tuna salad into lettuce leaves and wrap
   them up.

Spinach and Quinoa Stuffed Peppers

Ingredients:

- 4 bell peppers, halved and seeds removed
- 1 cup cooked quinoa
- 2 cups fresh spinach
- 1 can diced tomatoes, drained
- 1/2 cup shredded mozzarella cheese
- 1 teaspoon Italian seasoning
- Salt and pepper to taste

Instructions:

1. Preheat the oven to 375°F (190°C).

2. In a bowl, mix cooked quinoa, spinach, diced
   tomatoes, mozzarella cheese, Italian seasoning, salt,
   and pepper.

3. Fill each pepper half with the quinoa mixture.

4. Place stuffed peppers in a baking dish and cover with
   foil.

5. Bake for 25-30 minutes or until peppers are tender and filling is hot.

Chicken and Vegetable Stir-Fry

Ingredients:

- 2 boneless, skinless chicken breasts, sliced
- 2 cups mixed vegetables (bell peppers, broccoli, carrots)
- 2 cloves garlic, minced
- 2 tablespoons low-sodium soy sauce
- 1 tablespoon sesame oil
- 1 tablespoon honey
- 1 teaspoon ginger, grated
- Cooked brown rice for serving

Instructions:

1. In a wok or large skillet, heat sesame oil over medium-high heat.
2. Add chicken slices and cook until no longer pink.
3. Add minced garlic and ginger, stir for a minute.
4. Add mixed vegetables and cook until tender-crisp.
5. In a small bowl, mix soy sauce and honey.

6. Pour the sauce over the stir-fry and cook for a few more minutes.

7. Serve over cooked brown rice.

Greek Salad with Grilled Chicken

Ingredients:

- 2 boneless, skinless chicken breasts
- 6 cups mixed greens
- 1 cup cherry tomatoes, halved
- 1 cucumber, diced
- 1/4 cup red onion, thinly sliced
- 1/4 cup feta cheese
- Kalamata olives (optional)
- Greek dressing
- Salt and pepper to taste

Instructions:

1. Preheat a grill or grill pan over medium-high heat.

2. Season chicken breasts with salt and pepper.

3. Grill chicken until cooked through, about 6-7 minutes per side.

4. Let the chicken rest for a few minutes, then slice it.

5. In a large bowl, combine mixed greens, cherry tomatoes, cucumber, red onion, feta cheese, and olives (if desired).

6. Drizzle with Greek dressing and toss to coat.

7. Top with sliced chicken.

Veggie and Hummus Wrap

Ingredients:

- 4 whole-grain tortillas
- 1 cup hummus
- 2 cups mixed salad greens
- 1 bell pepper, thinly sliced
- 1 cucumber, thinly sliced
- 1 carrot, grated
- Salt and pepper to taste

Instructions:

1. Lay out a tortilla.

2. Spread a generous layer of hummus.

3. Add mixed salad greens, bell pepper, cucumber, and grated carrot.

4. Season with salt and pepper.

5. Roll the tortilla tightly, cut in half, and enjoy.

Bean and Vegetable Chili

Ingredients:

- 1 can low-sodium black beans, drained and rinsed
- 1 can low-sodium kidney beans, drained and rinsed
- 1 can low-sodium diced tomatoes
- 1 cup corn kernels
- 1 bell pepper, diced
- 1 onion, chopped
- 2 cloves garlic, minced
- 2 tablespoons chili powder
- 1 teaspoon cumin
- Salt and pepper to taste

Instructions:

1. In a large pot, sauté onion and garlic until softened.
2. Add beans, diced tomatoes, corn, and bell pepper.
3. Stir in chili powder and cumin.
4. Season with salt and pepper.
5. Simmer for 20-25 minutes.
6. Serve hot.

Turkey and Vegetable Stir-Fry

Ingredients:

- 2 boneless, skinless turkey breasts, sliced
- 2 cups mixed vegetables (bell peppers, broccoli, snap peas)
- 2 cloves garlic, minced
- 2 tablespoons low-sodium soy sauce
- 1 tablespoon sesame oil
- 1 tablespoon honey
- 1 teaspoon ginger, grated
- Cooked brown rice for serving

Instructions:

1. In a wok or large skillet, heat sesame oil over medium-high heat.
2. Add turkey slices and cook until no longer pink.
3. Add minced garlic and ginger, stir for a minute.
4. Add mixed vegetables and cook until tender-crisp.
5. In a small bowl, mix soy sauce and honey.
6. Pour the sauce over the stir-fry and cook for a few more minutes.
7. Serve over cooked brown rice.

Spinach and Mushroom Quesadilla

Ingredients:

- 2 whole-grain tortillas
- 2 cups fresh spinach
- 1 cup sliced mushrooms
- 1/2 cup low-fat shredded cheese
- 2 tablespoons olive oil
- Salt and pepper to taste

Instructions:

1. In a skillet, heat olive oil over medium heat.
2. Add mushrooms and sauté until tender.
3. Add spinach and cook until wilted.
4. Lay out a tortilla, sprinkle half of the cheese.
5. Add the spinach-mushroom mixture and top with the remaining cheese.
6. Place another tortilla on top.
7. Cook in a dry skillet until cheese is melted and tortillas are golden brown.
8. Slice and serve.

Cucumber and Chickpea Salad

Ingredients:

- 2 cups diced cucumber
- 1 can chickpeas, drained and rinsed
- 1/4 cup red onion, finely chopped
- 1/4 cup fresh parsley, chopped
- 2 tablespoons lemon juice
- 2 tablespoons olive oil
- Salt and pepper to taste

Instructions:

1. In a large bowl, combine diced cucumber, chickpeas, red onion, and parsley.
2. In a small bowl, whisk together lemon juice and olive oil.
3. Pour the dressing over the salad and toss to combine.
4. Season with salt and pepper.
5. Chill before serving.

Sweet Potato and Black Bean Salad

Ingredients:

- 2 cups sweet potato, diced and roasted
- 1 can black beans, drained and rinsed
- 1 red bell pepper, diced
- 1/4 cup red onion, finely chopped
- 1/4 cup cilantro, chopped
- 2 tablespoons lime juice
- 2 tablespoons olive oil
- Salt and pepper to taste

Instructions:

1. In a large bowl, combine roasted sweet potato, black beans, red bell pepper, red onion, and cilantro.
2. In a small bowl, whisk together lime juice and olive oil.
3. Pour the dressing over the salad and toss to combine.
4. Season with salt and pepper.
5. Serve chilled.

Caprese Salad with Balsamic Glaze

Ingredients:

- 4 ripe tomatoes, sliced
- 1 cup fresh mozzarella, sliced
- Fresh basil leaves
- Balsamic glaze
- Salt and pepper to taste

Instructions:

1. Alternate tomato, mozzarella, and basil slices on a serving plate.
2. Drizzle with balsamic glaze.
3. Season with salt and pepper.
4. Serve as a refreshing salad.

Lentil and Vegetable Curry

Ingredients:

- 1 cup red lentils
- 1 onion, chopped
- 2 cloves garlic, minced
- 1 can diced tomatoes

- 1 cup mixed vegetables (peas, carrots, bell peppers)
- 2 tablespoons curry powder
- 1 teaspoon cumin
- Salt and pepper to taste

Instructions:

1. In a large pot, sauté onion and garlic until softened.
2. Add lentils, diced tomatoes, mixed vegetables, curry powder, and cumin.
3. Season with salt and pepper.
4. Simmer for 20-25 minutes.
5. Serve hot over rice or with whole-grain naan.

Egg Salad Lettuce Wraps

Ingredients:

- 6 hard-boiled eggs, chopped
- 1/4 cup plain Greek yogurt
- 2 tablespoons Dijon mustard
- 2 tablespoons fresh dill, chopped
- Salt and pepper to taste
- Lettuce leaves for wrapping

Instructions:

1. In a bowl, combine chopped hard-boiled eggs, Greek yogurt, Dijon mustard, and fresh dill.

2. Mix well and season with salt and pepper.

3. Spoon the egg salad into lettuce leaves and wrap them up.

Zucchini Noodle Salad with Pesto

Ingredients:

- 2 zucchinis, spiralized into noodles
- 1/2 cup cherry tomatoes, halved
- 1/4 cup pine nuts
- 1/4 cup fresh basil leaves
- 1/4 cup grated Parmesan cheese
- Pesto sauce
- Salt and pepper to taste

Instructions:

1. In a large bowl, combine zucchini noodles, cherry tomatoes, pine nuts, basil leaves, and Parmesan cheese.

2. Drizzle with pesto sauce and toss to combine.

3. Season with salt and pepper.

4. Serve as a refreshing zucchini noodle salad.

Chapter 4: Dinner Recipes

In the quest for preparing wholesome and delicious dinners for those with dietary considerations, we bring you a selection of delectable recipes to tantalize your taste buds while adhering to a diabetic kidney-friendly meal plan. These recipes focus on fresh ingredients and flavors that make each dish not only nourishing but also incredibly satisfying.

Grilled Salmon with Lemon-Dill Sauce

Ingredients:

- 4 salmon fillets
- 2 tablespoons fresh lemon juice
- 1 tablespoon olive oil
- 1 teaspoon dried dill
- Salt and pepper to taste

Instructions:

1. Preheat your grill to medium-high heat.

2. In a bowl, combine lemon juice, olive oil, dried dill, salt, and pepper.

3. Brush the salmon fillets with the lemon-dill mixture.

4. Grill the salmon for about 4-5 minutes per side or until it flakes easily with a fork.

5. Serve with extra lemon-dill sauce drizzled over the top.

Baked Chicken Breast with Asparagus

Ingredients:

- 4 boneless, skinless chicken breasts
- 1 pound fresh asparagus
- 2 tablespoons olive oil
- 1 teaspoon garlic powder
- Salt and pepper to taste

Instructions:

1. Preheat your oven to 375°F (190°C).

2. Place chicken breasts and asparagus in a baking dish.

3. Drizzle with olive oil and season with garlic powder, salt, and pepper.

4. Bake for 25-30 minutes or until the chicken is cooked through.

Spaghetti Squash with Tomato Sauce

Ingredients:

- 1 medium spaghetti squash
- 2 cups sugar-free tomato sauce
- 1 teaspoon Italian seasoning
- Grated Parmesan cheese (optional)

Instructions:

1. Preheat your oven to 375°F (190°C).

2. Cut the spaghetti squash in half lengthwise and scoop out the seeds.

3. Place the squash halves face down in a baking dish with a little water.

4. Bake for 40-45 minutes until the flesh is tender and shreds like spaghetti.

5. Heat the tomato sauce, add Italian seasoning, and serve over the squash. Add Parmesan if desired.

Shrimp and Vegetable Skewers

Ingredients:

- 1 pound large shrimp, peeled and deveined
- Bell peppers, onions, and zucchini, cut into chunks
- Olive oil
- Garlic powder, paprika, and salt

Instructions:

1. Preheat your grill to medium-high heat.
2. Thread shrimp and vegetables onto skewers.
3. Brush with olive oil and season with garlic powder, paprika, and salt.
4. Grill for about 2-3 minutes per side or until shrimp turn pink and vegetables are tender.

Black Bean and Quinoa Stuffed Peppers

Ingredients:

- 4 large bell peppers
- 1 cup cooked quinoa
- 1 can black beans, drained and rinsed
- 1 cup salsa
- 1 teaspoon chili powder
- Shredded cheese for topping (optional)

Instructions:

1. Preheat your oven to 350°F (175°C).
2. Cut the tops off the bell peppers and remove the seeds.
3. In a bowl, mix cooked quinoa, black beans, salsa, and chili powder.
4. Stuff the peppers with the quinoa mixture.
5. Place stuffed peppers in a baking dish and cover with foil.
6. Bake for 25-30 minutes. If desired, remove foil and top with shredded cheese, then bake for an additional 5 minutes.

Garlic and Herb Roasted Turkey

Ingredients:

- 1 boneless turkey breast
- 2 tablespoons olive oil
- 3 cloves garlic, minced
- Fresh rosemary and thyme
- Salt and pepper

Instructions:

1. Preheat your oven to 325°F (165°C).
2. Rub the turkey breast with olive oil, minced garlic, fresh herbs, salt, and pepper.
3. Place it in a roasting pan.
4. Roast for about 1.5 to 2 hours or until the internal temperature reaches 165°F (74°C).

Tofu and Vegetable Stir-Fry

Ingredients:

- 1 block of firm tofu, cubed
- Mixed stir-fry vegetables

- Stir-fry sauce (low-sodium soy sauce, ginger, garlic, and honey)
- Cooked brown rice

Instructions:

1. Heat a pan, add tofu cubes, and stir until lightly browned.
2. Add mixed vegetables and stir-fry sauce.
3. Cook until veggies are tender.
4. Serve over cooked brown rice.

Grilled Swordfish with Mango Salsa

Ingredients:

- Swordfish steaks
- Olive oil
- Salt and pepper
- Mango, diced
- Red onion, diced
- Fresh cilantro

Instructions:

1. Preheat your grill to medium-high heat.

2. Brush swordfish with olive oil and season with salt and pepper.

3. Grill swordfish for about 4-5 minutes per side.

4. Combine diced mango, red onion, and cilantro to make a salsa.

5. Serve swordfish topped with mango salsa.

Cabbage and Sausage Skillet

Ingredients:

- 1 pound turkey sausage, sliced
- 1 head cabbage, shredded
- 1 onion, diced
- 2 cloves garlic, minced
- Salt and pepper to taste

Instructions:

1. In a large skillet, brown the turkey sausage.

2. Add diced onion and garlic, sauté until fragrant.

3. Stir in the shredded cabbage.

4. Cook, stirring occasionally, until the cabbage is tender.

5. Season with salt and pepper.

Baked Cod with Herb Crust

Ingredients:

- Cod fillets
- Olive oil
- Fresh herbs (thyme, rosemary, parsley)
- Garlic, minced
- Lemon juice

Instructions:

1. Preheat your oven to 375°F (190°C).
2. Brush cod fillets with olive oil and place them in a baking dish.
3. Mix fresh herbs, minced garlic, and lemon juice.
4. Sprinkle the herb mixture over the cod.
5. Bake for about 15-20 minutes or until the fish flakes easily.

Stuffed Zucchini Boats

Ingredients:

- Zucchinis, halved lengthwise
- Ground turkey or chicken

- Onion, diced

- Bell peppers, diced

- Tomato sauce

- Italian seasoning

Instructions:

1. Hollow out the zucchini halves.

2. In a pan, brown ground turkey or chicken with diced onion and bell peppers.

3. Mix in tomato sauce and Italian seasoning.

4. Stuff the zucchini halves with the meat mixture.

5. Bake for 20-25 minutes until the zucchini is tender.

Turkey and Vegetable Curry

Ingredients:

- Ground turkey

- Mixed vegetables

- Curry paste or powder

- Coconut milk

- Salt and pepper

Instructions:

1. In a pan, cook ground turkey.

2. Add mixed vegetables, curry paste or powder, and coconut milk.

3. Simmer until the vegetables are tender.

4. Season with salt and pepper.

Eggplant and Tomato Bake

Ingredients:

- Eggplants, sliced
- Tomatoes, sliced
- Olive oil
- Fresh basil leaves
- Parmesan cheese (optional)

Instructions:

1. Preheat your oven to 375°F (190°C).

2. Layer eggplant and tomato slices in a baking dish.

3. Drizzle with olive oil and sprinkle with fresh basil (and Parmesan if desired).

4. Bake for about 30 minutes until vegetables are tender and slightly browned.

Lemon Herb Tilapia

Ingredients:

- Tilapia fillets
- Lemon juice
- Fresh herbs (thyme, oregano, parsley)
- Garlic, minced
- Salt and pepper

Instructions:

1. Preheat your oven to 375°F (190°C).
2. Place tilapia fillets in a baking dish.
3. Drizzle with lemon juice and sprinkle with fresh herbs, minced garlic, salt, and pepper.
4. Bake for about 15-20 minutes or until the fish flakes easily.

Butternut Squash and Chickpea Stew

Ingredients:

- Butternut squash, cubed
- Chickpeas

- Onion, diced
- Garlic, minced
- Vegetable broth
- Curry powder

Instructions:

1. In a pot, sauté diced onion and minced garlic.
2. Add butternut squash, chickpeas, vegetable broth, and curry powder.
3. Simmer until the squash is tender.

Beef and Vegetable Stir-Fry

Ingredients:

- Lean beef strips
- Mixed stir-fry vegetables
- Stir-fry sauce (low-sodium soy sauce, ginger, garlic)
- Brown rice

Instructions:

1. Heat a pan, add beef strips, and stir-fry until browned.
2. Add mixed vegetables and stir-fry sauce.

3. Cook until veggies are tender.

4. Serve over cooked brown rice.

Mushroom and Spinach Stuffed Chicken

Ingredients:

- Chicken breasts
- Mushrooms, chopped
- Spinach, chopped
- Garlic, minced
- Olive oil
- Salt and pepper

Instructions:

1. Preheat your oven to 375°F (190°C).

2. In a pan, sauté mushrooms, spinach, and garlic in olive oil.

3. Slice a pocket into the chicken breasts and stuff with the mushroom-spinach mixture.

4. Bake for about 25-30 minutes or until chicken is cooked through.

Cilantro Lime Shrimp

Ingredients:

- Large shrimp, peeled and deveined
- Fresh cilantro
- Lime juice
- Garlic, minced
- Olive oil
- Salt and pepper

Instructions:

1. In a bowl, mix fresh cilantro, lime juice, minced garlic, olive oil, salt, and pepper.
2. Marinate the shrimp in this mixture for about 10 minutes.
3. Heat a pan and cook the shrimp until they turn pink and are cooked through.

Chapter 5: Snacks and Appetizers

When it comes to snacking and appetizers, finding options that are both delicious and health-conscious is crucial for anyone following a diabetic kidney-friendly meal plan. In this chapter, we've curated a diverse selection of snacks and appetizers that are not only easy to prepare but also packed with flavors and nutrients.

Mixed Nuts

Ingredients:

- 1/2 cup mixed nuts (almonds, walnuts, cashews)
- 1/2 teaspoon olive oil
- A pinch of sea salt

Instructions:

1. Preheat your oven to 350°F (175°C).
2. In a bowl, toss the mixed nuts with olive oil and a pinch of sea salt.
3. Spread the nuts on a baking sheet and roast for 10-15 minutes until lightly toasted.

4. Allow them to cool before serving.

Greek Yogurt and Berries

Ingredients:

- 1 cup Greek yogurt
- 1/2 cup fresh mixed berries (strawberries, blueberries, raspberries)
- 1 tablespoon honey (optional)

Instructions:

1. Place Greek yogurt in a serving bowl.
2. Top with fresh mixed berries.
3. Drizzle with honey if desired.

Hummus and Veggies

Ingredients:

- 1/2 cup hummus
- Assorted fresh veggies (carrots, cucumber, bell peppers)

Instructions:

1. Wash and cut the fresh veggies into sticks or slices.
2. Serve them with a bowl of hummus for dipping.

Cottage Cheese with Pineapple

Ingredients:

- 1/2 cup low-fat cottage cheese
- 1/2 cup pineapple chunks

Instructions:

1. Combine cottage cheese and pineapple chunks in a bowl.
2. Mix gently and enjoy.

Stuffed Bell Pepper Poppers

Ingredients:

- 3 bell peppers (red, yellow, or green)
- 1 cup cooked quinoa
- 1/2 cup black beans, drained and rinsed
- 1/2 cup corn kernels
- 1/2 cup diced tomatoes

- 1/4 cup shredded cheddar cheese
- 1 teaspoon chili powder
- Salt and pepper to taste

Instructions:

1. Preheat your oven to 350°F (175°C).
2. Cut the tops off the bell peppers and remove seeds and membranes.
3. In a bowl, mix cooked quinoa, black beans, corn, diced tomatoes, chili powder, salt, and pepper.
4. Stuff the bell peppers with the quinoa mixture.
5. Sprinkle shredded cheddar cheese on top.
6. Place the stuffed peppers in a baking dish and bake for 30 minutes or until the peppers are tender.

Guacamole with Veggie Sticks

Ingredients:

- 2 ripe avocados
- 1 lime, juiced
- 1 small red onion, minced
- 2 cloves garlic, minced
- 1-2 tomatoes, diced

- 1/2 teaspoon salt

- 1/4 teaspoon cayenne pepper (optional)

- Assorted veggie sticks for dipping (carrots, celery, cucumber)

Instructions:

1. In a bowl, mash the avocados with lime juice.
2. Stir in minced red onion, garlic, diced tomatoes, salt, and cayenne pepper.
3. Serve with veggie sticks.

Hard-Boiled Eggs

Ingredients:

- Eggs

Instructions:

1. Place eggs in a saucepan and cover them with water.
2. Bring the water to a boil, then reduce to a simmer.
3. Cook for 9-12 minutes for hard-boiled eggs.
4. Cool, peel, and enjoy.

Caprese Skewers

Ingredients:

- Cherry tomatoes
- Fresh mozzarella balls
- Fresh basil leaves
- Balsamic glaze

Instructions:

1. Thread cherry tomatoes, mozzarella balls, and fresh basil leaves onto skewers.
2. Drizzle with balsamic glaze.

Cucumber Slices with Tzatziki

Ingredients:

- 1 cucumber, thinly sliced
- 1 cup tzatziki sauce

Instructions:

1. Arrange cucumber slices on a plate.
2. Serve with tzatziki sauce for dipping.

Edamame

Ingredients:

- Edamame pods

Instructions:

1. Steam or boil edamame pods until tender.
2. Sprinkle with a pinch of sea salt and enjoy.

Apple Slices with Almond Butter

Ingredients:

- Apple slices
- Almond butter

Instructions:

1. Dip apple slices in almond butter for a delicious and nutritious snack.

Mini Turkey Lettuce Wraps

Ingredients:

- Ground turkey
- Lettuce leaves

- Sliced bell peppers
- Sliced carrots
- Hoisin sauce

Instructions:

1. Brown ground turkey in a pan.
2. Assemble lettuce wraps with turkey, bell peppers, carrots, and a drizzle of hoisin sauce.

Popcorn with Nutritional Yeast

Ingredients:

- Popcorn kernels
- Nutritional yeast
- Olive oil
- Salt

Instructions:

1. Pop popcorn according to package instructions.
2. Drizzle with olive oil, sprinkle nutritional yeast and salt for a savory snack.

Roasted Chickpeas

Ingredients:

- Canned chickpeas, drained and rinsed
- Olive oil
- Seasonings (e.g., paprika, cumin, salt)

Instructions:

1. Toss chickpeas with olive oil and seasonings.
2. Roast in the oven at 400°F (200°C) until crispy.

Mini Caprese Salad

Ingredients:

- Cherry tomatoes
- Fresh mozzarella balls
- Fresh basil leaves
- Balsamic glaze

Instructions:

1. Assemble cherry tomatoes, mozzarella balls, and basil leaves.
2. Drizzle with balsamic glaze.

Sliced Bell Peppers with Peanut Butter

Ingredients:

- Sliced bell peppers
- Peanut butter

Instructions:

1. Dip bell pepper slices in peanut butter for a unique and tasty combination.

Baked Sweet Potato Fries

Ingredients:

- Sweet potatoes, cut into fries
- Olive oil
- Paprika
- Salt

Instructions:

1. Toss sweet potato fries with olive oil, paprika, and salt.
2. Bake in the oven at 425°F (220°C) until crispy.

Rice Cake with Avocado

Ingredients:

- Rice cakes
- Ripe avocados
- Salt and pepper

Instructions:

1. Spread mashed avocado on rice cakes.
2. Season with salt and pepper for a satisfying snack.

Chapter 6: Desserts

In this delectable section, we delve into the world of sugar-free desserts designed to satisfy your sweet cravings while keeping your blood sugar in check. These desserts are not just guilt-free but also bursting with flavor. Whether you have a penchant for fruity treats or crave chocolatey indulgence, there's something here to please every palate.

Sugar-Free Berry Sorbet

Ingredients:

- 2 cups of mixed berries (strawberries, blueberries, raspberries)
- 1 tablespoon of fresh lemon juice
- 1/4 cup of water
- Stevia or your preferred sugar substitute (to taste)

Instructions:

1. Blend the mixed berries, lemon juice, and water until smooth.

2. Add your chosen sweetener gradually, adjusting to your desired level of sweetness.

3. Pour the mixture into a container and freeze for at least 3 hours.

4. Scoop and enjoy a refreshing berry sorbet.

Chocolate Avocado Pudding

Ingredients:

- 2 ripe avocados
- 1/4 cup of unsweetened cocoa powder
- 1/4 cup of almond milk
- Stevia or your preferred sugar substitute (to taste)
- 1 teaspoon of vanilla extract

Instructions:

1. Scoop out the flesh of the avocados and place it in a blender.

2. Add cocoa powder, almond milk, sweetener, and vanilla extract.

3. Blend until the mixture is smooth and creamy.

4. Refrigerate for about 30 minutes before serving.

Baked Apple with Cinnamon

Ingredients:

- 2 apples
- 1/2 teaspoon of ground cinnamon
- A drizzle of honey (optional)

Instructions:

1. Preheat your oven to 350°F (175°C).
2. Core the apples and place them in a baking dish.
3. Sprinkle cinnamon over the apples.
4. Drizzle with honey if desired.
5. Bake for 30-40 minutes or until the apples are tender and aromatic.

Greek Yogurt Parfait with Honey

Ingredients:

- 1 cup of Greek yogurt
- 1/2 cup of mixed berries
- 1 tablespoon of honey (or a sugar substitute)

Instructions:

1. In a glass or bowl, start with a layer of Greek yogurt.
2. Add a layer of mixed berries.
3. Drizzle honey (or a sugar substitute) on top.
4. Repeat the layers as desired.
5. Garnish with extra berries and a drizzle of honey.

Frozen Banana Bites

Ingredients:

- 2 bananas
- 1/4 cup of dark chocolate chips (sugar-free)
- 1/4 cup of chopped nuts (e.g., almonds, walnuts)

Instructions:

1. Slice the bananas into bite-sized pieces.
2. Melt the dark chocolate chips in the microwave or over a double boiler.
3. Dip each banana slice into the melted chocolate.
4. Roll the chocolate-covered banana in chopped nuts.
5. Place on a baking sheet and freeze for about 2 hours.

Chia Seed Chocolate Pudding

Ingredients:

- 3 tablespoons of chia seeds

- 1 cup of almond milk

- 2 tablespoons of unsweetened cocoa powder

- Stevia or your preferred sugar substitute (to taste)

- 1/2 teaspoon of vanilla extract

Instructions:

1. In a bowl, mix chia seeds, almond milk, cocoa powder, sweetener, and vanilla extract.

2. Stir well, and let it sit in the fridge for a few hours or overnight.

3. Enjoy the chocolatey chia pudding.

Berry and Almond Tart

Ingredients:

- 1 cup of almond flour

- 2 tablespoons of coconut oil

- Stevia or your preferred sugar substitute (to taste)

- 1 cup of mixed berries

Instructions:

1. Combine almond flour, coconut oil, and sweetener to form a crust.
2. Press the crust into a tart pan or individual tartlet molds.
3. Fill the tart with mixed berries.
4. Refrigerate until firm, then serve.

Oatmeal Raisin Cookies (Sugar-Free)

Ingredients:

- 1 cup of rolled oats
- 1/2 cup of raisins
- 1/2 cup of almond flour
- 1/4 cup of unsweetened applesauce
- Stevia or your preferred sugar substitute (to taste)

Instructions:

1. Preheat the oven to 350°F (175°C).
2. In a bowl, mix oats, raisins, almond flour, applesauce, and sweetener.

3. Drop spoonfuls of the mixture onto a baking sheet.

4. Bake for 12-15 minutes or until the cookies are golden.

Pumpkin Pie Smoothie

Ingredients:

- 1/2 cup of canned pumpkin (unsweetened)
- 1/2 cup of almond milk
- 1/2 teaspoon of pumpkin pie spice
- Stevia or your preferred sugar substitute (to taste)
- Ice cubes

Instructions:

1. Blend the canned pumpkin, almond milk, pumpkin pie spice, sweetener, and ice cubes until smooth.

2. Adjust sweetness to your liking.

3. Serve the smoothie in a chilled glass.

Lemon Blueberry Muffins (Sugar-Free)

Ingredients:

- 1 cup of almond flour
- 1/2 cup of blueberries
- 2 tablespoons of lemon juice
- Stevia or your preferred sugar substitute (to taste)
- 1/2 teaspoon of baking powder

Instructions:

1. Preheat your oven to 350°F (175°C).
2. In a bowl, combine almond flour, blueberries, lemon juice, sweetener, and baking powder.
3. Mix well and spoon the batter into muffin cups.
4. Bake for 20-25 minutes or until the muffins are lightly browned.

Almond and Coconut Bites

Ingredients:

- 1/2 cup of almond butter
- 1/4 cup of shredded coconut

- Stevia or your preferred sugar substitute (to taste)
- 1/2 teaspoon of vanilla extract

Instructions:

1. In a bowl, mix almond butter, shredded coconut, sweetener, and vanilla extract.
2. Form the mixture into bite-sized balls.
3. Refrigerate for an hour to firm them up.

Avocado Chocolate Mousse

Ingredients:

- 2 ripe avocados
- 1/4 cup of unsweetened cocoa powder
- Stevia or your preferred sugar substitute (to taste)
- 1 teaspoon of vanilla extract

Instructions:

1. Scoop out the flesh of the avocados and place it in a blender.
2. Add cocoa powder, sweetener, and vanilla extract.
3. Blend until the mixture is smooth and creamy.
4. Refrigerate for about 30 minutes before serving.

Peach and Raspberry Crumble

Ingredients:

- 2 cups of sliced peaches
- 1 cup of fresh raspberries
- 1/2 cup of almond flour
- Stevia or your preferred sugar substitute (to taste)

Instructions:

1. Preheat your oven to 350°F (175°C).
2. In a baking dish, combine the peaches and raspberries.
3. In a separate bowl, mix almond flour and sweetener.
4. Sprinkle the almond flour mixture over the fruit.
5. Bake for 25-30 minutes until the topping is golden.

Rice Pudding with Cinnamon

Ingredients:

- 1/2 cup of cooked brown rice
- 1 cup of unsweetened almond milk
- Stevia or your preferred sugar substitute (to taste)
- 1/2 teaspoon of ground cinnamon

Instructions:

1. In a saucepan, combine cooked rice, almond milk, sweetener, and cinnamon.

2. Cook over low heat, stirring occasionally, until the mixture thickens.

3. Serve warm or chilled, sprinkled with extra cinnamon.

Strawberry Cheesecake Bites

Ingredients:

- 1 cup of fresh strawberries
- 4 oz of cream cheese (reduced-fat)
- Stevia or your preferred sugar substitute (to taste)
- 1/2 teaspoon of vanilla extract

Instructions:

1. Remove the tops from the strawberries and scoop out the center to create a small cavity.

2. In a bowl, mix cream cheese, sweetener, and vanilla extract.

3. Fill each strawberry with the cheesecake mixture.

Carrot Cake Bites

Ingredients:

- 1 cup of shredded carrots
- 1/2 cup of almond flour
- Stevia or your preferred sugar substitute (to taste)
- 1/2 teaspoon of cinnamon

Instructions:

1. In a bowl, combine shredded carrots, almond flour, sweetener, and cinnamon.
2. Form the mixture into bite-sized balls.
3. Refrigerate for an hour to firm them up.

Apple Cinnamon Baked Oatmeal

Ingredients:

- 1 cup of rolled oats
- 1 apple, diced
- 1/2 teaspoon of ground cinnamon
- Stevia or your preferred sugar substitute (to taste)
- 1 cup of almond milk

Instructions:

1. Preheat your oven to 350°F (175°C).

2. In a baking dish, mix rolled oats, diced apples, cinnamon, sweetener, and almond milk.

3. Bake for 25-30 minutes or until the top is golden and the oats are cooked.

Peanut Butter Protein Balls

Ingredients:

- 1/2 cup of natural peanut butter
- 1/2 cup of protein powder (choose a sugar-free variety)
- Stevia or your preferred sugar substitute (to taste)

Instructions:

1. In a bowl, combine peanut butter, protein powder, and sweetener.

2. Form the mixture into small balls.

3. Refrigerate for an hour before enjoying these protein-packed treats.

CONCLUSION

As we wrap up this journey through the world of diabetic kidney-friendly meal planning, it's essential to reflect on the profound impact your choices can have on your health. This chapter serves as a reminder that this is not just about following a set of recipes but embracing a lifestyle that promotes well-being.

In these pages, we've explored the intricacies of crafting meals that cater to your specific dietary needs. Yet, it's crucial to understand that this is not the end but the beginning of a new chapter in your life. The conclusion here is merely a transition, not a final destination.

Maintaining a Healthy Diabetic Kidney-Friendly Lifestyle:
This section underscores that the principles you've learned are not limited to the pages of this guide. They should permeate your daily life, becoming ingrained in your choices and habits. It's about making conscious decisions to protect your health.

Final Thoughts and Encouragement:

Your health journey can be challenging, and it's perfectly okay to face setbacks and doubts. In this part of the chapter, we offer words of encouragement. Remember that every small step you take towards a healthier lifestyle is a victory. Stay motivated and know that you have the power to make a difference in your health.

In summary, this chapter, like the broader journey, is about empowerment. It's about taking control of your health and well-being, one meal at a time. You are the author of your story, and this guide is just one tool in your arsenal. As you move forward, keep your health as a priority, and let it be the guiding star in your life's narrative.